FOOD POISONING

TACTICAL WAYS OF DEALING WITH FOOD
POISONING

DR. ULRIC WALSH

Contents

CHAPTER ONE

INTRODUCTION

Food poisoning, a kind of foodborne infection, is a contamination human beings get from some thing they ate or drank. The causes are germs or one-of-a-kind risky topics within the meals or beverage.

Symptoms of meals poisoning frequently include disenchanted stomach, diarrhea and vomiting. Symptoms and signs usually begin inside hours or numerous days of eating the meals. The general public have moderate contamination and get higher with out remedy.

Once in a while meals poisoning reasons

intense contamination or complications.

Meals poisoning or foodborne contamination can arise to absolutely everyone who swallows inflamed food. The general public get better on their very very own, but some can grow to be gravely sick. You're more at risk in case you are pregnant, older than sixty five or have a weakened immune system. More youthful kids also are greater at hazard, especially from dehydratlon.

Meals poisoning, or foodborne infection, takes place whilst you consume infected food. Inflamed technique it's infected with a toxic organism, together with a bacteria, fungus, parasite or virus. Once in a while the poisonous byproducts of these organisms purpose meals poisoning.

When you consume some component poisonous, your frame reacts to purge the toxins. You can purge via vomiting, diarrhea, fever or all of those. The uncomfortable symptoms of meals poisoning are your frame's manner of working to go back to fitness. It usually works in a day or .

Food poisoning (foodborne infection) is as a result of bacteria or viruses observed in food.

Food poisoning is an contamination you get from consuming food that has micro organism, a pandemic, or a parasite in it.

Signs

Symptoms vary counting on what is causing the contamination. They'll begin within a few hours or a few weeks counting on the purpose.

Not unusual signs and symptoms are:

Disillusioned belly.

Vomiting.

Diarrhea.

Diarrhea with bloody stools.

Stomach pain and cramps.

Fever.

Headache.

Lots less regularly meals poisoning impacts the tense device and might motive immoderate sickness. Signs and symptoms might also consist of:

Blurred or double imaginative and prescient.

Headache.

Loss of motion in limbs.

Problems with swallowing.

Tingling or numbness of pores and skin.

Weak point.

Modifications in sound of the voice.

What's the difference among meals poisoning and belly flu?

Meals poisoning and belly flu are each gastrointestinal infections. They each cause gastroenteritis, that's contamination of your stomach and small intestine. Gastroenteritis is the signal that your immune machine has been activated to remove the infection.

Among the equal viral, bacterial and other infections can reason food poisoning or belly flu, resulting within the same signs and signs and symptoms. The principle distinction is that foodborne infection comes from food, whilst you can trap a stomach bug in a spread of other ways.

How will you inform if it's food poisoning or some thing else?

It is able to be tough to tell in which an contamination got here from, specifically if it took a few days to develop signs. You'll be able to trace it decrease lower back to some aspect you ate if it became some thing normally associated with meals poisoning, or if you have been with a person else who additionally got ill.

What motives food poisoning?

Maximum meals poisoning is on account of eating meals that has positive kinds of micro organism or viruses. At the same time as you consume those food, the micro organism maintains growing on your digestive tract. This reasons an infection.

Meals also can make you sick in the event that they have a toxin or poison made with the resource of micro organism growing in the food.

Several sorts of micro organism can reason food poisoning. The numerous greater common bacteria are:

Salmonella and Campylobacter

Can be observed in meat, chicken, and eggs

which might be raw or not cooked prolonged enough (undercooked)

May be found in dairy products that haven't long gone thru a high-warmth method to kill micro organism (are unpasteurized)

May be decided in raw culmination and greens

Clostridium perfringens

May be found in uncooked meat, chicken, eggs, or unpasteurized dairy ingredients

Can be found in greens and plants which have touched soil

Can cause meals poisoning when soups, stew, and gravies made with meat, fish, or chicken aren't refrigerated

Listeria

Can be determined in unpasteurized milk and gentle cheeses made with unpasteurized milk

Can also be located in deli meats, warm dogs, and store-made deli salads

Staphylococcus aureus

Can unfold to meals whilst touched by way of way of someone with the bacteria

Can cause contamination while ingredients which includes meats and egg salad aren't refrigerated

Escherichia coli (E. Coli)

Can purpose contamination if you devour

pork that is undercooked, especially floor beef

May be determined in unpasteurized milk

Can be observed in meals or water this is contaminated

You could additionally get food poisoning from viral ailments which include Hepatitis A. The ones viral diseases:

Can bypass from an infected person's hands to the arms of food workers or into waste water (sewage)

Can unfold at the same time as shellfish and exclusive foods have touched dangerous, dirty water

Botulism is a rare however lethal shape of food poisoning. It is as a result of a micro organism (clostridium botulinum) this is decided for the duration of, even in soil and water.

You devour low-acid meals that are not properly canned or preserved at home. Those components encompass meat, fish, bird, or vegetables.

Infants consume uncooked honey or corn syrup. Toddlers more younger than 1 12 months vintage should in no manner have honey or corn syrup.

Whilst to look a physician

Infants and youngsters

Vomiting and diarrhea can rapid purpose low ranges of frame fluids, additionally known as dehydration, in toddlers and youngsters. This could reason excessive illness in infants.

Call your toddler's health care provider in case your little one's signs embody vomiting and diarrhea and any of the following:

Unusual adjustments in behavior or thinking.

Immoderate thirst.

Little or no urination.

Vulnerable factor.

Dizziness.

Diarrhea that lasts greater than an afternoon.

Vomiting frequently.

Stools that have blood or pus.

Stools which can be black or tarry.

Intense pain within the belly or rectum.

Any fever in children below 2 years of age.

Fever of 102 ranges Fahrenheit (38.Nine tiers Celsius) or higher in older kids.

Information of different scientific issues.

Adults

Adults ought to see a health care issuer or get emergency care if the following arise:

Apprehensive machine symptoms, which include blurry imaginative and prescient, muscle weak point and tingling of pores and skin.

Changes in thinking or behavior.

Fever of 103 ranges Fahrenheit (39.4 tiers Celsius).

Vomiting regularly.

Diarrhea that lasts more than three days.

Signs and signs and symptoms of dehydration — excessive thirst, dry mouth, little or no urination, intense weak point, dizziness, or lightheadedness.

Who receives meals poisoning?

Definitely anybody can get meals poisoning if they devour inflamed food. However a few people are more likely to get ill from infection than others. It has to do with how an awful lot toxicity your body can typically tolerate without getting unwell.

Our immune systems constantly fend off infections with out our understanding approximately it. Even with sanitary food managing practices, there is often a small amount of contamination in our meals. It becomes "poisonous" even as our immune systems attain their threshold.

Who's maximum at chance from foodborne contamination?

You'll be much more likely to get unwell from meals poisoning, or have a more extreme response to food poisoning, if your immune system isn't as sturdy as common. Quick subjects can impact your immunity, in addition to longer-term conditions, in conjunction with:

Age. Kids below the age of five have immature immune structures. Mature immune structures begin to decline after the age of 65.

Pregnancy. Pregnancy is disturbing at the body, leaving you with fewer belongings than ordinary to combat off infections.

Continual illnesses. Many continual conditions can have an effect on your immunity, which include infections, maximum cancers, immunodeficiency sicknesses and autoimmune ailments.

Medications. Corticosteroids and immunosuppressants can repress your immune machine and make you greater at risk of infection.

CHAPTER TWO

How is meals poisoning identified?

Your healthcare business enterprise will ask you even as you became sick, what your signs are, and what foods you have got got eaten.

Your issuer can even have a look at your beyond health. He or she will give you a physical examination.

You can have lab checks to discover what bacteria added about your infection. In a few instances the motive can't be located.

Headaches

In maximum wholesome adults,

complications are unusual. They can encompass the subsequent.

Dehydration

The most commonplace problem is dehydration. This a excessive lack of water and salts and minerals. Both vomiting and diarrhea can reason dehydration.

Maximum wholesome adults can drink sufficient fluids to save you dehydration. Youngsters, older adults, and people with weakened immune structures or other ailments might not be capable of update the fluids they've got out of place. They are much more likely to become dehydrated.

Individuals who end up dehydrated can also need to get fluids straight away into the bloodstream at the clinic. Excessive dehydration can purpose organ damage, different extreme ailment and loss of life if now not treated.

Complications of systemic disorder

Some contaminants can motive greater big sickness within the body, additionally called systemic ailment or infection. That is greater commonplace in folks who are older, have weakened immune structures or different medical conditions. Systemic infections from foodborne bacteria might also additionally motive:

Blood clots in the kidneys. E. Coli can bring about blood clots that block the kidneys' filtering device. This condition, referred to as hemolytic uremic syndrome, consequences in the sudden failure of the kidneys to filter waste from the blood. A whole lot less often, other micro organism or viruses may additionally motive this situation.

Micro organism in the bloodstream. Micro organism inside the blood can purpose sickness within the blood itself or unfold disease to other components of the body.

Meningitis. Meningitis is infection that can harm the membranes and fluid surrounding the mind and spinal cord.

Sepsis. Sepsis is an overreaction of the immune tool to systemic sickness that damages the body's own tissues.

Pregnancy headaches

Contamination from the listeria bacteria within the route of pregnancy can bring about:

Miscarriage or stillbirth.

Sepsis inside the new infant.

Meningitis in the newborn.

Rare headaches

Uncommon headaches encompass conditions that can increase after food poisoning, which encompass:

Arthritis. Arthritis is swelling, tenderness or ache in joints.

Irritable bowel syndrome. Irritable bowel syndrome in a lifelong state of affairs of the intestines that reasons ache, cramping and ordinary bowel movements.

Guillain-Barre syndrome. Guillain-Barre syndrome is an immune tool attack on nerves that could result in tingling, numbness and loss of muscle manipulate.

Breathing troubles. Rarely, botulism can damage nerves that manage the muscle mass concerned in respiratory.

Remedies for food Poisoning

Some treatments for meals poisoning ease the signs, on the identical time as others help to prevent dehydration, which can make signs and symptoms worse.

Resting Your body

Easy rest is one way to assist your frame

heal from food poisoning. Take it clean until you sense higher.

Moreover, do no longer consume or drink for some hours after the onset of symptoms and signs and symptoms. While you do start eating and drinking once more, strive slight and bland food, like crackers, and sports activities drinks. Suck on ice chips to live hydrated.

Hydrating With Electrolytes

One of the most commonplace complications of any foodborne contamination is dehydration, especially among younger youngsters and older adults. The scenario may be lethal if it's now not treated right away.

Dehydration because of commonplace signs and symptoms of meals poisoning — diarrhea and vomiting — can motive you to lose hundreds of fluid in a short time. A lack of fluids inside the body can reason tiredness, vulnerable factor, and every so often even abnormal heartbeats.

Except the dehydration is severe, it's often treatable at home and consistent with your physician's commands. Sports activities beverages or water with electrolyte pills can commonly ease moderate dehydration. Serious cases may additionally want to necessitate going to a clinic or health center at once to get intravenous (IV) fluids right now into your frame thru your veins.

Following the BRAT weight loss plan

The BRAT diet is mild at the belly and consists of bananas, rice, applesauce, and toast. Eat this for so long as you're now not feeling well. You could also encompass clean broths in this eating regimen.

This weight loss program includes food that assist make your stools more impregnable and helps to fill up nutrients you could have lost all through your contamination. If you pick not to study this food regimen, ensure to consume smaller and coffee-fats meals till you're feeling better.

Along with Probiotics to your food

Probiotics are organisms that help to keep your gut biome in take a look at. Each person has micro organism living internal of them all the time. A number of these are "right micro organism," and a few are "awful bacteria."

Food poisoning can throw off the sensitive stability of remarkable and awful bacteria for your intestine. Taking probiotics can convey it lower returned into balance. They'll additionally give a boost to your gut to protect you from future foodborne infection.

Over-the-counter drug remedies may also prevent the signs and signs and symptoms of food poisoning. Bismuth subsalicylate — you can apprehend this medication as Pepto-Bismol — can deal with nausea and diarrhea. Loperamide — you can understand this as

Imodium — is an antidiarrheal that stops diarrhea through slowing down the digestive technique.

It's critical to note that those products are typically not meant for youngsters, but. The meals and Drug administration (FDA) recommends that younger children with diarrhea drink fluids and observe their ordinary healthy dietweight-reduction plan, even though food regimen modifications and rehydration answers can be needed if the hassle maintains.

A few docs say that the usage of over the counter medicinal drugs may additionally assist you heal quicker. However, distinct docs say that it may be higher to allow the contamination run its path without preventing nausea and diarrhea with over the counter remedies.

Drinking Ginger or Mint Tea

Ginger root is a staple in conventional medication practices of multiple cultures. Studies display that it does relieve nausea oftentimes.

Mint is likewise an herb that traditional remedy practitioners say can settle the belly. It may have a pain-relieving software precise to the intestine. Drinking tea also can assist you live hydrated while you are sick.

Prevention

To prevent meals poisoning at domestic:

Handwashing. Wash your palms with soap and water for at least 20 seconds. Do that after using the toilet, before consuming, and earlier than and after managing meals.

Wash culmination and vegetables. Rinse stop end result and veggies underneath walking water before eating, peeling or getting geared up.

Wash kitchen utensils thoroughly. Wash slicing forums, knives and one of a kind utensils with soapy water after contact with uncooked meats or unwashed give up result and greens.

Do not devour uncooked or undercooked meat or fish. Use a meat thermometer to make certain meat is cooked sufficient. Put together dinner entire meats and fish to at least 145 F (63 C) and let rest for at least three mins. Put together dinner ground meat to at the least 160 F (seventy one C). Prepare dinner whole and floor bird to at least one hundred sixty five F (seventy four C).

Refrigerate or freeze leftovers. Placed leftovers in blanketed packing containers inside the fridge right after your meal. Leftovers can be stored for 3 to four days inside the refrigerator. In case you do no longer assume you may eat them inside 4 days, freeze them proper away.

Prepare dinner leftovers efficiently. You may safely thaw frozen food three strategies. You may microwave it. You could skip it to the fridge to thaw in a single day. Or you could placed the frozen food in a leakproof container and positioned it in cold water at the counter. Reheat leftovers until the internal temperature reaches one hundred sixty five degrees Fahrenheit (74 levels Celsius).

Throw it out whilst uncertain. If you aren't certain if a meals has been prepared, served or saved adequately, discard it. Even though it looks and smells awesome, it can no longer be safe to devour.

Throw out moldy food. Throw out any baked elements with mold. Throw out moldy mild fruits and vegetables, including tomatoes, berries or peaches. And throw away any nuts or nut merchandise with mildew. You may trim away mildew from organisation elements with low moisture, which consist of carrots, bell peppers and tough cheeses. Reduce away as a minimum 1 inch (2.Five centimeters) around the moldy part of the meals.

Smooth your fridge. Smooth the interior of the refrigerator every few months. Make a cleaning solution of one tablespoon (15 milliliters) of baking soda and 1 quart (zero.Nine liters) of water. Clean visible mold in the fridge or on the door seals. Use a solution of one tablespoon (15 milliliters) of bleach in 1 quart of water.

Safety for at-chance humans

Food poisoning is particularly important all through pregnancies and for younger kids, older adults and people with weakened immune structures. The ones illnesses may be existence-threatening. Those people should avoid the following elements:

Raw or undercooked meat, hen, fish, and shellfish.

Uncooked or undercooked eggs or substances that could consist of them, along with cookie dough and selfmade ice cream.

Uncooked sprouts, which consist of alfalfa, bean, clover and radish sprouts.

Unpasteurized juices and ciders.

Unpasteurized milk and milk products.

Gentle cheeses, along side feta, brie and Camembert; blue-veined cheese; and unpasteurized cheese.

Refrigerated pates and meat spreads.

Raw heat puppies, luncheon meats and deli meats.

Conclusion

Even in present day, evolved international locations in which food handling practices are fantastically sanitary, meals poisoning still normally takes place. You may be even extra at danger in case you travel overseas. For the most element, our immune structures are nicely-prepared to deal with the occasional contamination.

But, nice infections can purpose intense aspect effects, mainly in the more prone amongst us. If you are concerned or immunocompromised, or when you have intense or uncommon symptoms and symptoms, do now not hesitate to peer your healthcare provider for checking out and treatment.

THE END

www.ingramcontent.com/pod-product-compliance
Lightning Source LLC
Chambersburg PA
CBHW060820260726
48660CB00003B/1018